Contents

Understanding CBD

CBD stands for cannabidiol. It is one of 113 cannabinoids that's found in cannabis. It is non-addictive and also non-psychoactive. CBD is extracted from the cannabis plant during production and is separated from the THC, which is the psychoactive element of cannabis. Cannabidiol (CBD) is one of many cannabinoids that can be found in hemp and marijuana, two types of cannabis plants.

CBD may help people with cancer manage some symptoms of the disease as well as side effects of treatment. Scientists are also looking into how CBD could aid cancer treatment, but more research is needed before any conclusions can be made.

Marijuana has enough tetrahydrocannabinol (THC) to get you high, but hemp does not. CBD itself has no psychoactive compounds

CBD oil has garnered a reputation as being an effective treatment for neurological and physiological illnesses. People who use CBD oil love that it's a natural product that is generally much easier on the body when compared to most pharmaceuticals. It's commonly used to treat pain, anxiety, and insomnia, but can CBD oil work for cancer patients?

Those that want to seek the supposed relief that cannabis may provide, may now seek it through the use of CBD. Those suffering from anxiety, depression, pain, cancer, and other ailments are turning to CBD for the possible relief and bodily equilibrium that it may provide. There are not any known health risks associated with CBD… however; those taking certain medication should proceed with caution. In any case, we recommend consulting with a medical professional for those who take medication which may interact with grapefruit (Read more about CBD drug interactions here. In fact, there are innumerable reports throughout common widespread media that attribute CBD to its' positive prophylactic effects

This book will take an in-depth look at everything you need to know about using CBD for cancer treatment.

How Are CBD Products Made?

Many people know that CBD comes from cannabis. It's right there in the name: cannabidiol.

But, how exactly does CBD oil get made? What happens in the transition from the hemp plant to a product you can buy online or in your local health store?

All CBD products contain CBD oil, which is extracted from the hemp plant. This is why you'll often see "hemp extract" on the label and in the ingredients list. After extraction, the oil is added to various products, including CBD oil tinctures, gummies, capsules, topicals, and vape oils.

CBD Extraction Methods

When people talk about how CBD products are made, they're mainly talking about the specific extraction method. The most common methods to extract CBD oil use carbon dioxide, steam distillation, or hydrocarbon or natural solvents. We review each of these below.

Carbon Dioxide (CO2) Extraction

CO2 extraction uses supercritical carbon dioxide to separate the CBD oil from the plant material. "Supercritical" refers to the CO2 containing properties of both a liquid and a gas state, which is why you'll sometimes see this method referred to as Supercritical Fluid Extraction (SFE).

During CO2 extraction, a series of pressurized chambers and pumps are used to expose CO2 to high pressure and very low temperatures, resulting in an extracted oil containing high amounts of CBD.

At the start of extraction, one chamber will hold pressurized CO_2, while a second pressurized chamber holds the hemp plant.

The CO_2 is then pumped from the first chamber into the second. The presence of supercritical CO_2 breaks down the hemp also in the chamber, causing the oil to separate from the plant material.

Finally, the CO_2 and oil are pumped together into a third chamber. The gas evaporates, leaving an extract of pure CBD oil behind.

While it requires expensive specialized machinery, CO_2 extraction is the preferred method for making CBD products. It's extremely safe and efficient at producing high concentrations of CBD in the resulting oil—as much as 92% according to one analysis.

Carbon dioxide extraction for CBD oil

The precise nature of CO_2 extraction also makes it suitable for producing specific concentrations of CBD oil. Manufacturers can simply adjust the solvent and pressure ratios to achieve the desired concentration of CBD.

The CO2 extraction process is also widely used to create many other products besides CBD oil, such as decaffeinating coffee or tea, or extracting essential oils for use in perfumes.

Steam Distillation

With steam distillation, steam causes the CBD oil to separate from the hemp plant. The hemp plant is contained in a glass flask, with an inlet and an outlet. The inlet connects to another glass container, beneath the plant flask, that contains water that is set to boil. The outlet connects to a condenser tube.

Steam distillation for cbd

As the water heats up, the steam travels upwards into the plant flask, separating the oil vapors that contain CBD.

These vapors are then captured in a tube that condenses them into oil and water.

Once collected, the oil and water mixture is distilled to extract the CBD oil from the water.

The steam distillation technique is tried and true, having been used to extract essential oil for centuries, but it's less preferred than CO_2 extraction due to its inefficiency. Steam distillation requires significantly larger amounts of hemp plant, and it's more difficult to extract exact amounts of CBD concentration using this method.

There's also an element of risk with this method. If the steam gets too hot, it can damage the extract and alter the chemical properties of the cannabinoids it contains.

Solvent Extraction (Hydrocarbons and Natural Solvents)

Solvent extraction follows a similar process to steam distillation, except that it uses a solvent rather than water to separate the CBD oil from the plant material. This creates a resulting mixture of the CBD oil with the solvent. The solvent then evaporates leaving pure CBD oil behind. Solvent extraction uses either hydrocarbons or natural solvents.

Solvent extraction is more efficient than steam distillation, and it's also less expensive. However, the solvents used in hydrocarbon extraction (including naphtha, petroleum, butane, or propane) create cause for concern. The solvent residue can be toxic and increase one's cancer risk if they aren't fully eliminated during the evaporation step—which doesn't always happen. Some studies have found traces of petroleum or naphtha hydrocarbons residue in CBD products that used solvent extraction.

To avoid the risk of toxic residue, solvent extraction can use natural solvents instead, such as olive oil or ethanol. These solvents are just as effective at extracting CBD oil, but remove the risk of toxic residue.

However, natural solvent extraction is not without its downsides. When natural solvents like ethanol are used, chlorophyll may also be extracted. This gives the resulting oil an unpleasant taste. If the CBD is used in capsules or topicals, this isn't a big deal, but many CBD products are eaten or inhaled (such as gummies, tinctures, vape oils), so this can make them harder to sell.

The larger problem with natural solvents, though, is that they don't evaporate very well. As a result, the CBD extract contains a lower concentration of CBD than it would with other methods.

What Is the Best Extraction Method for CBD Oil?

There are pros and cons to each extraction method. At CBDOil.org, we recommend CO2 extraction. While it is the most expensive extraction method, it consistently produces the highest concentration of CBD, resulting in a □uality product.

It's also one of the safest extraction methods, leaving behind no neurotoxic residue.

Extraction Method Pros Cons

CO2 Extraction Efficient

Highest concentration of CBD

Easier to adjust concentration

No toxic residue

No chlorophyll Expensive

Steam Distillation Inexpensive

No toxic residue

No chlorophyll Inefficient

12

Inconsistent concentration of CBD

Potential for heat to damage CBD oil

Hydrocarbon Solvent Extraction Efficient

Inexpensive

Consistent concentration of CBD

No chlorophyll Potential for toxic solvent residue

Natural Solvent Extraction Efficient

Inexpensive

No toxic residue Presence of chlorophyll affects taste

Lower concentration of CBD

When purchasing CBD products, find out which extraction method the company uses, as this can be an indicator of the □uality and value of their products. Products that use CO2 extraction may be more expensive, but they also tend to be higher-□uality.

CBD products made using other extraction methods can be safe and high-□uality as well, but there can be more risk with these products. Specifically, CBD products that were made using hydrocarbon extraction may contain solvent residuals. And while steam distillation and natural solvent extraction are lower-risk, they can produce lower or inconsistent amounts of CBD, which can affect the cost/mg value of your CBD product.

Beyond their extraction method, also confirm that the company uses a third-party lab to test the concentration of the CBD in their products, as well as the safety of the other ingredients. Any reputable manufacturer will make these test results readily available on their website, with their product packaging, or upon request. The test results will show the potency of the CBD and other cannabinoids (described in milligrams). They'll also reveal any potential contaminants, as well as the presence of any solvent residue, if the product used hydrocarbon solvent extraction.

What Happens After Extraction?

After extraction, the resulting CBD oil is described as "full-spectrum." This means that other cannabinoids besides CBD, including CBDA, CBDV, THC, and others, are still present. As long as the product is sourced from hemp, the amount of THC will be 0.3% or less (which makes it legal anywhere in the U.S.).

Full-spectrum CBD oils also contain other beneficial elements from the plant material, such as terpenes and amino acids. Many people prefer full-spectrum CBD oil because of the "entourage effect." While this effect has not been proven, some users believe that the CBD is able to engage the endocannabinoid system more effectively when more cannabinoids are present.

However, some people would rather have no THC in their oil, even in very low, legal amounts. These people prefer CBD isolates. To create CBD isolate, the extract is cooled and further purified into crystalline isolate form. This results in a white, flavorless powder. Because it contains only CBD, CBD isolate is less expensive per milligram, contains no THC, and has no flavor or odor.

Finally, regardless of whether it is turned into a CBD isolate or remains full-spectrum, the CBD oil is added to other substances to create various CBD products.

The CBD may be mixed with a carrier oil like hemp seed oil or coconut oil to create CBD oil tinctures.

To create CBD gummies, the CBD oil may be combined with natural flavoring, juice, and organic corn syrup.

The CBD oil may be mixed with a variety of ingredients to create CBD edibles like baked goods or chocolates.

With CBD capsules, the CBD oil is often added to MCT oil (a coconut oil extract) to give the capsule volume. If it's a softgel, the capsule may also use olive oil to create the casing.

To create CBD vape oils, the CBD oil is combined with a mix of vegetable glycerin and propylene glycol (to make it suitable for inhalation) and natural flavoring (for better taste).

The CBD oil may be combined with various essential oils, shea butter, aloe vera, and waxes to create CBD creams, skin salves, and other topicals.

Can CBD be used as a complementary cancer therapy?

Cancer is an extremely complicated disease. It affects organs and areas throughout the body. As a result, the treatment plans for each cancer can differ, but studies have shown that CBD may help treat cancer alongside other treatment options. In particular, it can help with stimulating appetite, pain relief, and nausea.

Stimulating appetite – Cancer treatment can be extremely tough on your body. Chemotherapy and intense medication can make it difficult to have an appetite. Some patients lose lots of weight during their treatment, but tests have shown that CBD can stimulate appetite in children.

Pain relief – CBD has been shown to be an effective way to deal with pain. It inhibits the CB2 receptor in the brain which helps to reduce inflammation. Pain and inflammation can come from the cancer itself and also from cancer treatment. So using CBD for cancer treatment may be an effective relieve option for patients.

Nausea – Chemotherapy is a necessary evil for some patients. It can help destroy the cancer cells, but it can also come with some extreme side effects. Nausea is a common side effect associated with chemotherapy and for some, it can be devastating. Tests have shown that CBD can help reduce chemotherapy-induced nausea.

CBD may work as an effective complement to traditional cancer therapy, but does it work as a treatment for cancer?

Cancer treatments such as chemotherapy and radiation can produce an array of side effects, such as nausea and loss of appetite, which can lead to weight loss. Research suggests that cannabinoids may ease neuropathic pain, nausea, and poor appetite due to cancer and cancer treatment. CBD is also thought Trusted Source to have anti-inflammatory and anti-anxiety properties.

So far, only one CBD product has received Food and Drug Administration (FDA) approval Trusted Source. That product is Epidiolex, and its only use is in the treatment of two rare forms of epilepsy. No CBD products have been FDA-approved to treat cancer or symptoms of cancer, or to ease side effects of cancer treatment.

On the other hand, two marijuana-based drugs have been approved to treat nausea and vomiting caused by chemotherapy. Dronabinol (Marinol) comes in capsule form and contains THC. Nabilone (Cesamet) is an oral synthetic cannabinoid that acts similar   to   THC.

Another cannabinoid drug, nabiximols, is available in Canada and parts of Europe. It's a mouth spray containing both THC and CBD and has shown promise in treating cancer pain. It's not approved in the United States, but it is the subject of ongoing research.If you're considering using medical marijuana, talk to your doctor about how best to administer it. Smoking may not be a good choice for people with certain types of cancer.

CBD and other cannabis products come in many form, including vape, tincture, sprays, and oils. It can also be found in candies, coffee, or other edibles.

CBD for cancer treatment

Studies into whether or not CBD can treat the cancer cells themselves rather than acting as a complementary treatment are still in their early days. More tests are needed to reach definite conclusions, but some of the early results are positive.

According to a test in 2019, cannabinoids can have positive effect on pancreatic cancer. It was shown to help slow tumor growth and invasion, while even inducing tumor cell death.

CBD was also shown to make glioblastoma cells more sensitive to radiation, without damaging healthy cells.

It seems that CBD is a good complementary therapy and potentially even a treatment for cancer, but can it prevent cancer?

A 2019 review of in vitro and in vivo studies focusing on pancreatic cancer found that cannabinoids can help slow tumor growth, reduce tumor invasion, and induce tumor cell death. The study authors wrote that research into the effectiveness of different formulations, dosing, and precise mode of action are lacking and urgently needed.A 2019 study trusted Source indicated that CBD could provoke cell death and make glioblastoma cells more sensitive to radiation, but with no effect on healthy cells.

A large, long-term study trusted Source of men within the California Men's Health Study cohort found that using cannabis may be inversely associated with bladder cancer risk. However, a cause and effect relationship hasn't been established. A 2014 study in experimental models of colon cancer in vivo suggests that CBD may inhibit the spread of colorectal cancer cells.

A review Trusted Source of 35 in vitro and in vivo studies found that cannabinoids are promising compounds in the treatment of gliomas.

Other research demonstrated the efficacy of CBD in pre-clinical models of metastatic breast cancer. The study found that CBD significantly reduced breast cancer cell proliferation and invasion.

These are just a few studies addressing the potential of cannabinoids to help treat cancer. Still, it's far too soon to say that CBD is a safe and effective treatment for cancer in humans. CBD shouldn't be considered a substitute for other cancer treatment.

Some areas for future research include:

➢ The effects of CBD with and without other cannabinoids like THC
➢ Safe and effective dosing
➢ The effects of different administration techniques
➢ How CBD works on specific types of cancer
➢ How CBD interacts with chemotherapy drugs and other cancer treatments

CBD Oil for cancer prevention?

This particular application of CBD needs much more research. There have been no tests that showed CBD to be an effective cancer prevention method. These tests take a long time and must consider variables such as dosing, types of cancer, types of patients and other medication used.

As a result, CBD is currently not considered to be an option for cancer prevention. However, CBD may sound like a great option for people who are currently diagnosed with cancer, but are there any side effects?

Studies on the role of cannabinoids in the development of cancer have produced mixed resultsTrusted Source.

A 2010 study using a mouse model found that cannabinoids can trigger suppression of the immune system. That could make users more susceptible to some types of cancer. This particular research involved cannabis containing THC.When it comes to cancer prevention, CBD research has a long way to go. Scientists will have to conduct long-term studies of people using specific CBD products, controlling for frequency of use, dosing, and other variables.

Side effects

As with most medical products, there can be some side effects. Side effects can happen if you take too large of a dose. Your body composition and metabolism levels can also affect how your b The World Health Organization (WHO)Trusted Source says that CBD has a good safety profile and that negative side effects may be due to interactions with other medications. It states that there's no evidence of public health-related problems from the use of pure CBD.

In 2017, a large review of studies Trusted Source found that CBD is generally safe, with few side effects. Among them are:

- ➢ Appetite changes, which could be a good thing for people in cancer treatment
- ➢ Diarrhea
- ➢ Tiredness
- ➢ Weight changes

More research is needed to understand other effects of CBD, such as whether it affects hormones. Researchers also want to know more about how CBD may increase or decrease the effects of other medications. The review does suggest some concern that CBD may interfere with liver enzymes that help metabolize certain medications. That could lead to higher concentrations of these medications in the system.

CBD, like grapefruit, interferes with the metabolizing of certain medications. Talk to your doctor before using CBD, especially if you take a medication that comes with a "grapefruit warning" or one of the following:

- ➢ Antibiotics
- ➢ Antidepressants or anti-anxiety medications

> Antiseizure medications
> Blood thinners
> Muscle relaxers, sedatives, or sleep aids
> Oral or IV chemotherapy

The American Cancer Society supports the need for more research on cannabinoids for cancer patients.ody deals with CBD.

Brief explanation of these effects:

> **Diarrhea** – Patients have noted that diarrhea is a side effect associated with CBD. This is believed to occur when taking very large doses. If you experience this side effect either lower your dose or speak with your doctor to make sure you're on the correct dosage. It is believed that the carrier oil of the CBD upsets the gastrointestinal tract which can cause diarrhea.

> **Tiredness** – CBD is used as a natural sleep remedy, so it's no surprise that it can cause tiredness and drowsiness

in patients. These feelings can last between two and six hours. This side effect can be dealt with by taking the CBD oil at night rather than during the day. If you suffer from tiredness after taking CBD oil it is very important that you do not drive.

➢ **Appetite change** – CBD can affect people in different ways. Some CBD oil users have noticed an increase in their appetite, while others have noted a decrease in appetite. For cancer patients having an increase in appetite may be a good thing. This will encourage you to eat more and get more vitamins and nutrients into your body.

➢ **Weight changes** – As with any change in your appetite, you may also notice changes in weight. Nausea may make eating seem uninviting but cancer patients are encouraged to maintain a healthy weight to help beat cancer. If CBD oil prevents you from eating and makes you lose weight then you may need to change your dose or find alternative methods.

Side effects with CBD oil are generally less common and less severe than traditional pharmaceuticals. As it is extracted from the cannabis plant which is still listed as a Class B Drug it raises the question, is CBD oil safe?

Is it safe?

CBD oil is widely considered safe to use. Experts believe that it is near impossible to overdose on CBD. There have been no recorded deaths anywhere in the world that has been attributed to CBD. It is non-addictive and for most, side effects can be resolved by altering the dosage or method of consumption.

CBD is also non-psychoactive. One of the main concerns coming from people who are new to CBD is that it will get them high and make them hallucinate. CBD oil will not make you high. THC is the psychoactive component of cannabis that will get you stoned. For a CBD product to be legally sold in the UK it must have a THC level of 0.3% or less.

Now that you know that CBD oil can be used for cancer patients, what is the best way to use it?

How to use CBD oil

CBD oil can be used in a number of ways. This helps to make it a viable option for many cancer patients. Some methods take longer to enter the bloodstream while others have no taste and can be taken discreetly.

If patients are going to use CBD, ensure the product they use is free from contaminants, is third party tested, and they are communicating their use with providers to check for any potential drug-drug interactions.

It is possible that CBD could have a benefit with symptoms of anxiety, poor sleep, and pain. CBD has been studied a lot in the laboratory and in mice but far less in humans. Right now there are some studies that are evaluating CBD as a part of cancer treatment, but none of those have had significant results. The studies that do show a benefit with CBD are for specific epilepsy syndromes in children.

Capsules – Capsules are a good starting point for people who may be wary of side effects or worried about getting the exact dose. CBD capsules come with an exact dose of CBD in them. This dose should be clearly labelled on the bottle. Cancer patients may find using capsules as an easy way to integrate CBD into their lives as they will be already taking other forms of medication.

Vaping – Vaping has become a very popular way to consume CBD. The CBD is infused into an e-liquid that is then used with a normal vaping pen. Smoking is a well known carcinogenic so cancer patients are obviously advised to not smoke. Vaping is an option for people who are trying to overcome a smoking addiction as currently, there is no evidence to suggest that vaping directly causes cancer. Vaping CBD can help alleviate some of the pain associated with cancer.

Tinctures – CBD oil tinctures are probably what you imagine when you think of CBD oil. It comes in a glass bottle and has a handy dropper to help select the correct dose. CBD tinctures can be easily integrated into your daily life. Some like to drop the CBD oil directly under their tongue, while others like to add it to a drink or their food.

Edibles – Many people will imagine 'pot brownies' when they think of edibles, but there is now a huge market for CBD edibles. CBD is infused with gummies, lollipops and other treats. This is a great way to discreetly consume some pre-dosed CBD.

What does the research say?

The world of medicinal cannabis and CBD seems to be changing every day. With government writing new laws for cannabis use and public perception changing, researchers are now intensely investigating the medical applications of CBD. To get conclusive results a lot of time and money is needed because of this, research is still at a very early stage. Early signs are promising in a lot of areas, but it is still too early to say for sure that CBD is a successful form of cancer treatment on its own.

Tests have shown that CBD may be effective against some forms of breast cancer. In pre-clinical models of metastatic breast cancer tests have shown that CBD reduced breast cancer cell proliferation and invasion. CBD also performed well when tasked with treating gliomas, which are a type of brain tumors, in vitro and in vivo studies.

Future tests plan to investigate how CBD works with specific types of cancers and how it interacts with chemotherapy drugs. This current lack of scientific answers has resulted in people turning towards anecdotal evidence.

However, limited critical human trials on which cancers respond to the treatment of cannabinoids has slowed down the process of getting cannabinoids on the list of official cancer treatment options.

While cannabinoids are far from being considered a treatment for cancer, it has certainly proven to be successful in treating many forms of cancer as well as potentiating the effects of chemotherapy. As studies continue to be intensified, there is light at the end of the tunnel.Those that want to seek the supposed relief that cannabis may provide, may now seek it through the use of CBD. Those suffering from anxiety, depression, pain, cancer, and other ailments are turning to CBD for the possible relief and bodily equilibrium that it may provide. There are not any known health risks associated with CBD... however; those taking certain medication should proceed with caution. In any case, we recommend consulting with a medical professional for those who take medication which may interact with grapefruit. In fact, there are innumerable reports throughout common widespread media that attribute CBD to its' positive prophylactic effects

Anecdotal evidence

We've all heard stories of how CBD has helped out in individual cases. While these stories can't be accepted as a scientific fact, they can give hope that one day the full effect of CBD will be known.

Lynn Cameron from the UK was given 18 months to live in 2013. She had an aggressive form of brain cancer and doctors told her that she was terminally ill. Chemotherapy and radiation were not working for her and around that time a friend of hers told her to try CBD oil. She was put off by the fact that it was illegal at that time but decided to try it anyway. She began taking CBD oil daily and at every subsequent scan, Lynn had a reduction in tumor size. After the sixth MRI scan, the cancer had gone.

Anecdotal evidence must be taken with a grain of salt. If you have any questions please speak to your doctor for the latest information regarding using CBD for cancer. If you do decide to use CBD oil it is important to get the dosage right. Our next section discusses how to do that.

CBD dosage guide for cancer

The typical method of finding a possible CBD dosage is to start off with a miniscule amount. For instance, users might start off with 3-5 mg dosage for the first week. If the user experiences no change, they might increase to 10 mg, and continue increasing it bit by bit until they find it subjectively effective and consistent in providing possible relief.

Take into account the condition or symptoms you're trying to treat. From chronic pain to glaucoma to epilepsy to sleep disorders, there are plenty of different conditions that may require different dosage levels. If your symptoms cause severe pain, seizures, or other extreme symptoms, higher dosages may be necessary. We have taken this into account during the construct of our CBD Dosage Calculator. Our estimation calculator allows our users to select an ailment and the associated severity where applicable in order to better estimate a starting and goal dosage of CBD…

There is no exact formula to work out the dosage for individuals. Instead, a number of factors are considered to estimate a good starting point. From there, patients can adjust their dosage depending on their needs and their reaction to the CBD.

It is advised that you speak with your doctor and allow them to recommend a starting dose. The doctor will take a variety of things into consideration, including your weight, body composition, the type of cancer present and how CBD interacts with your current medication.

Once you have the recommended dose you may have a bit more work to do. Capsules and edibles all come pre-portioned with exact doses, but for CBD oil tinctures you will need to figure out how many drops is equal to your dose. If you have a 10 ml bottle of CBD oil it will contain 200 drops as one drop is 0.05 ml. That means that in a bottle with 1000 mg of CBD each drop will have 5 mg of CBD.

Here are some of the different methods of using CBD, as well as some pros and cons you might want to consider before choosing the method that works for you.

Tincture: This can come in drop or spray form which is delivered directly into the mouth. This is the most widely advocated, and the easiest to control the dose of. However, not all bottles display the per dose amount, so choose carefully.

This method is the most popular method of CBD consumption. Because it comes in liquid form, users appreciate the ease of quantifying and measuring the proper dosage for their ailments. Sublingual application is the typical method utilized with tinctures.

Tinctures are capable of carrying the most amount of CBD per volume versus the other methods of CBD.

Topical: These are balms or body rubs, which are considered as possibly the safest and most cautious way to use CBD. However, a lot of it is needed to provide an effective dose, which can make it very expensive to use. The dose is never precise because it is "eye balled".

Edibles: From foodstuffs like gummies and muffins to pills, finding CBD-enhanced foods or pills is relatively easy, and it's certainly the tastiest way to ingest it. However, it also takes much longer to absorb since it has to go through your digestive system before it ends up in the bloodstream. Some edibles are not able to carry adequate dosages.

Vape pens: While these are the fastest form of delivering CBD into the bloodstream and are easy to use, it is also very difficult to control your dosage, given how easy it is to continuously use vape pens.

One form may be more effective for you than others, so the fact that you might not find edibles or topicals effective does not mean that CBD doesn't necessarily work for you. If you want to control your dosage levels, however, tinctures are the most recommended form.

Conclusion

So is CBD oil a viable option for cancer patients? We know that CBD can be used as a complementary treatment alongside medication and chemotherapy. It's great for alleviating pain and nausea associated with traditional cancer treatments. However, scientists are still unsure as to whether or not CBD can actually help prevent cancer.

If you decide to use CBD you have a wide variety of ways to use it. Make sure that you speak with a medical professional first and be aware of the potential side effects.

However, limited critical human trials on which cancers respond to the treatment of cannabinoids has slowed down the process of getting cannabinoids on the list of official cancer treatment options.

If patients are going to use CBD, ensure the product they use is free from contaminants, is third party tested, and they are communicating their use with providers to check for any potential drug-drug interactions.

www.ingramcontent.com/pod-product-compliance
Lightning Source LLC
Chambersburg PA
CBHW030543220526
45463CB00007B/2960